Copyright Info
Disclaimer
Dedication
Acknowledgements
My Image
Introduction My Story
Chapter 1 The Missing Fluff
Chapter 2 Attempts with No Success
Chapter 3 Overview of the Process
Chapter 4 Step by Step
Images of my mole removal process
Chapter 5 Some Final Thoughts
About the Author
Publisher Info

Disclaimer

No part of this publication may be reproduced in any form or by any means, including printing, scanning, photocopying, or otherwise without the prior written permission of the author or publisher.

All content within this publication is commentary or opinion and is protected under Free Speech laws in the entire civilized world. This publication and its content is provided for educational and entertainment purposes only. Please note anything said in this book is NOT a substitute for medical advice.

The author and publisher assumes no responsibility for any errors, omissions, or contrary interpretation of the subject matter present in this publication. The author and the publisher shall have neither liability nor responsibility to any person or entity with respect to any loss, damage, or injury caused or alleged to be caused directly or indirectly by the information contained in this publication.

The information presented herein is in no way intended as a substitute for medical advice or medical attention. Always CONSULT YOUR DOCTOR.

Dedication

This book is dedicated to all of you who suffer with moles and took it upon yourselves to see what could be done about it. Those who don't seek answers are resigning themselves to the status quo..

I would like to dedicate this to my wife who puts up with me as I get wild ideas and dig and search and experiment with the answers. You are an amazing woman my Love, I'm a blessed man to have you in my life!

Love you Sweetheart!

Acknowledgements

Thank you to so many that put bits, pieces and breadcrumbs out there for me to follow. They allowed me to come up with my own solution that changed my appearance by removing those large moles from my face, and completely rebuilt how I saw myself. These generous few empowered me to pay it forward and share the solutions that worked for me with others to hopefully help them on their own journey.

To my wife, Lisa, who was invaluable, supportive, who encouraged me, put up with me and took this raw information and helped shape it into something that was understandable, without her this would not have been possible.

To Blair, who helped me find my way out of a very dark place, to move forward, while regaining myself. He set some stakes in the ground and got me to move past them with this book. Thank you!

Introduction
My Story

My name is Milo, and I have had my own personal experiences with Moles for most of my adult life. I thought I would share these experiences with the hopes that some of you would find the answers you are seeking.

I was a programmer and Unix system administrator for a large gaming company before developing an autoimmune disease: multiple sclerosis. The diagnosis was devastating and it changed the trajectory of my life and forced me to look at things differently. I wasn't satisfied with the "medical" options I was given, and it led me to seek alternative remedies.

In addition to my autoimmune disease I had another major problem. This problem was moles. I don't have just a few moles, I have tons of them (100's) most were flat and on my arms, legs, torso, and even my ears. I also developed a set of moles on my face—several became very large—and I felt self-conscious about them.

Now picture yourself with several very large moles on your face, prominent and sticking out. How would your reaction be to meeting people or going to the store? I felt ugly, powerless and ashamed. Every time I was going to meet someone it was at the forefront of my mind. I couldn't comprehend why this had to happen to me on top of my autoimmune disease. The other moles I have bother me too but clothing covers up the majority of them. The ones on my face however were going to be making that first impression before I ever spoke a word. To me it singled me out, basically saying "something wrong here".

More importantly, I didn't want to have them continue to grow, and I especially didn't want people to feel uncomfortable around me. It is possible that I made a bigger deal about this in my head than in reality, but I know people noticed, and I was embarrassed by it.

I didn't want to feel ugly to my wife or daughter and didn't want them embarrassed being seen with me. I know that isn't how they viewed me, and yet part of me still ran this through my mind constantly.

This all came to a head one week after a man stopped me in a store and told me I had a form of elephantiasis. That made my day! I understood where he was coming from because he said he had it too and had several large moles on his face.

I don't have elephantiasis; neither did the man who stopped me. Elephantiasis is a symptom of a variety of diseases, where parts of a person's body swell to massive proportions. But it really got me thinking that it was time I did something about this. The final nudge over the edge was a little later that same week. I was at a gathering with kids, and we all know how much filter kids can use. None. One little girl looked up at me and asked, "what's wrong with your face"? I didn't have an answer for her. But I knew in that moment that I didn't want moles to be a part of my life any more. I knew I had to do something.

I spoke to doctors about my moles. They either wanted to freeze and / or cut them out. I didn't want scarring and the other issues that come along with doing that. I seriously debated to go ahead and do it anyway, but a voice in me thought there had to be something else I could try first.

Because of my ability to treat my autoimmune disease with results that seemed to confound the doctors, I tried to find a more natural way of dealing with the moles. I searched the net, the library, talked with people, purchased books, purchased systems and did the good old trial and error to find out what worked for me. I know everyone is different, but I hope those reading will find the information I share—the information contained in this book—to be invaluable. The process that worked for me took years to discover and refine.

When I successfully removed the moles from my face, it was as if a huge weight was lifted off my shoulders. I didn't realize how much I had become withdrawn from others. People I knew were complimenting me. Asking me things like "did you lose weight? You look good, what have you changed?" Most didn't equate it to the moles, because they were gone, but they recognized that there had been some obvious changes in my life.. My wife and daughter, to my appreciation, told me it made me look younger as well..

I got my self-confidence back.

Best of all, not only did I get rid of them, but I REMOVED THEM. I made it happen, I figured it out.

After my transformation, I got inquiries on how I accomplished all of this, and it led to me sharing my story here.

At the outset, I want to explain that I am not a doctor, and this book is not giving you medical advice. I am simply sharing my personal experiences on what I did to get rid of moles from my body. This book is for informational purposes only.

I would recommend that you have your moles medically evaluated. There are good reasons to have your moles checked out by a medical doctor. These can include seeing if anything is abnormal with your moles or requires special attention.

Chapter 1
The Missing Fluff

This is a short chapter.

When I first started planning out this book, I had planned to write all about moles. Provide you with knowledge that I had tracked down about various types of moles and how they are caused. I would then paraphrase the information in a way those of us without medical degrees could understand. I found that in reality it seemed more that moles, -happen-. I couldn't find a WHY that the moles were forming. What I usually found is that the cells cluster instead of spread out and those cells give skin their color. Not really the why they were doing that, but its the how. The technical details are best left up to those institutions that specialize in that information. I would spend a little while doing some reading utilizing search engines for what causes moles, types of moles, how moles form, why do I have moles, etc.

I thought I could have chapters filled with this information. I thought about what I would have personally liked when I started this, what I would have liked to read. I decided I wanted to focus on what I did to get rid of my moles, without filling in a lot of fluff that was better served elsewhere.

Chapter 2
Attempts with No Success

I have a wide variety of different types of moles. I have a lot of moles all over my body (100's of them). I needed something that was effective in treating them. The types I removed from my face were raised moles as you can see from the images I've included.

As I've mentioned, the moles I was most self conscious about were the ones that appeared on my face. Sometimes someone would stare at me or I would get asked about them.

After talking to the doctors and hearing their solutions of freezing, burning, or cutting, I made a personal decision that I didn't want the potential scarring those procedures would leave behind.. Besides, it was fairly costly, to have 5-7 moles removed was more money than I could afford.

I saw a number of products advertised on the Internet. I didn't have much luck with them. It doesn't mean they don't work, it's just they didn't work for me and were quite expensive.

I tried mineral oil and baking soda, I tried Oregano oil, and this might have worked except the scent was so strong you couldn't even be around yourself, or others. It's possible some of these might have worked if I had figured out the emery board method, which I will talk about later. I didn't go back and try them. You'll see why.

An Important word about one thing that did happen that I want to share. It is what happened when I attempted to remove a flat mole, (like a very big freckle). That did not go well, it burned/stung a bit and settled into a scar area about the size of the freckle.

Chapter 3
Overview of the Process

I will walk you through an overview of the entire process, including both the successes and failures and what worked better as my path of discovery took me forward.

Prepping the Mole

The first thing I found with my failures was that the Mole had to be roughed up. Initially I tried to scrape it with a needle, that didn't seem to work too well.

I was using sewing needles, sterilized them by first burning the tip with a lighter, and then used alcohol to wipe it off. I then tried to poke the mole with the needle, but it was frankly too big. I then tried a much smaller needle, like the type used for insulin pens. These would poke through easily and I would pincushion the mole from the top several times and around the sides. This method led to my first sign of it working.

I thought that the needle poking would hurt, but as long as I didn't push the needle past where the 'normal' skin layer was under the mole, I felt nothing. I just had to be careful. I guess the mole doesn't seem to have any nerve endings itself, which in retrospect makes sense.

After using needle method to remove several of the moles, I discovered using an emery board was more effective. Using an emery board to rough up the skin all the way around and across the top was much more effective, seemed more sane, and sped up the process.

When using the needle method I had to keep re-poking the skin every time I applied product until it started the breakdown process. I found that using an emery board started that process much more quickly.

Protecting the Surrounding Skin

When using the emery board I was careful not to scratch the skin around the mole. I would gather my supplies and get prepared. I sometimes would put coconut oil, or petroleum Jelly lightly on the skin surrounding the mole to protect it. I was careful, however, not to get any of these products on the mole itself.

The Application

I cut a cotton ball down to a reasonable size, poured out my Apple Cider Vinegar (I used an organic brand my store carried called Braggs.) Putting on gloves, I would then soak the cotton ball, squeezing out the excess, but keeping it wet. I would start the timer on my phone for 20 minutes. I would wrap the mole in the flattened wet cotton ball, keeping firm pressure but not squeezing to make it difficult to hold for the allotted time. I would refresh the cotton ball in the Apple Cider Vinegar from time to time during the twenty minutes. If the mole were small or difficult to get to (like one I had on my nose or in my eyebrow) I would use a cotton swab. I would let it air dry at first eventually placing a drop of Apple Cider Vinegar on an adhesive bandage and placing it on there. The mole would crust or scab and with successive soaking they would fall off. I continued this till the mole was completely gone. It was at times ugly to look at a gooey mess, but they became little scabs that went away and left no mole or scar.

I have illustrated the process in a step-by-step fashion, but with warning that pictures are graphic.

Chapter 4
Step by Step Process

Let me start by showing you my face with my moles. I will begin with the two largest moles, one on each side of my face about the size of my pinky. You'll notice that they are very predominate and noticeable. The next picture displays what they looked like after I removed them. These moles were my first successes and I learned more as I continued to remove other moles.

Before Image

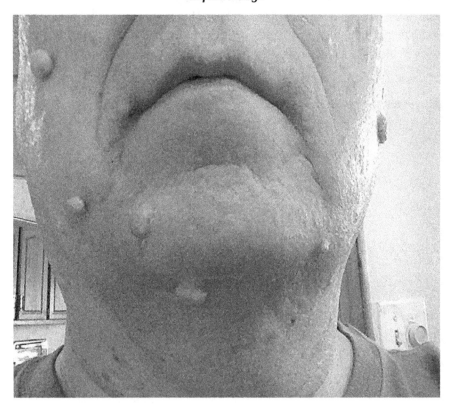

After Image

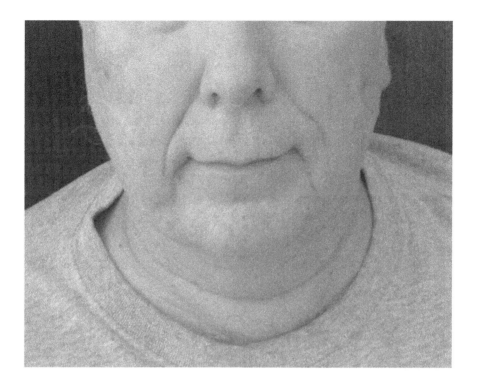

Supplies that I used:

- Emery board, thin needle - The first item is an emery board (yes, like you used to shape your nails). I also used a needle at first but found the emery board worked better for me. For a needle I actually used a very thin type used for insulin injections. I believe technically it is referred to as a 30 gauge
- Cotton balls or flat cotton pads (real cotton not synthetic). I eventually switched to the cotton pads, usually 50 or 100 in flat packs, because they were much easier to use and held more liquid.
- Disposable latex gloves, or food service gloves
- Cotton Swab
- Paper towel
- A timer (I used the timer on my phone)
- Adhesive bandages, large enough to cover the mole.
- A bottle of Apple Cider Vinegar - I used Braggs Organic Apple
- Cider Vinegar with the "Mother." (ACV for short) I like the Bragg's

brand.
- A small bowl (a disposable one is fine)
- Petroleum Jelly or Coconut Oil (to protect the surrounding skin)

Prep:

I would take the cotton ball and cut it into a size that when wet will still cover the entire mole. For me this typically meant cutting it in half and cutting one of those halves in half again. This is about a quarter of a cotton ball. I moved from the cotton balls to the cotton pads and would do the same, cutting it in half twice, depending on the size of the mole. It needs to be able to cover my mole when it was wet and flattened out.

Roughing it up:

This is where I would scratch, rough or poke the surface of the mole.

I started doing this step because just applying product didn't seem to do anything. Doing this seems to allow the surface of the mole to be penetrated with what we were going to be doing later in the process.

There were two ways I did this.

My first moles that I successfully removed I use the needle to attempt to scratch the surface and then discovered that I could just simply poke into the mole itself. This was not painful as long as I did not poke on the mole into the skin layer below. I would poke on the top and the sides penetrating the mole multiple times. I use this method for three of the moles on my face. I found I had to use the needle several times at the beginning of the mole remove until it started being affected and started to break down. It would require several sessions until it started showing signs of being affected. As mentioned, the emery board worked better as I only did this a couple of times until it started to show that it was working.

The remaining facial moles I used the emery board and simply scratched and roughed the entire surface of the mole.

I found using the emery board method was simpler and seemed to be more effective. I included the needle poking method in case you are having difficulty in the effectiveness of the scratching method.

Step One:

I discovered that for some moles, I wanted to protect the surrounding skin. The ACV can irritate and can cause chafing or burning on the surrounding skin. I carefully put on Coconut (or Petroleum Jelly) on the skin surrounding the mole without applying any to the mole itself.

Step Two:

I would shake up the apple cider vinegar; pour a small amount of the apple cider vinegar into a small bowl (enough to soak a cotton ball in several times over the 20 minutes).

Step Three:

I wore gloves, as I did not want to soak my fingers in apple cider vinegar for a long period of time.

Take your cotton ball or cotton pad and cut it into a size that when wet will still cover the entire mole. For me this typically meant cutting it in half and cutting one of those halves in half again. This is about a quarter of a cotton ball or pad.

Dip the quarter cotton ball or pad in the apple cider vinegar and flatten it gently squeezing out most of the liquid. You still want to keep it slightly wet just not dripping (you're not going to be ringing it out).

I found the cotton pads worked the best once I started using them.

Step Four:

While I did not find this step very painful, there was occasionally a little sting.

With the flat apple cider soaked cotton ball or pad, I would wrap around and hold tight the mole covering as much as possible to the base of the mole.

I needed to be careful here, as I did not want to dribble or drip ACV on my skin. I would have a paper towel ready to wipe anything that ran down. When I did this—if I noticed that the skin around my mole was getting irritated—I would take to applying a little coconut oil or petroleum jelly on the skin before I applied the Apple Cider Vinegar to the mole itself. I would be extra careful not to get coconut oil or petroleum jelly on the mole itself because that would protect the mole from the ACV.

I would hold the mole for 20 minutes (I wore gloves on both hands so I could switch). I would refresh the apple cider vinegar on the cotton wrap periodically during this time.

Step Five:
My first moles I did not bandage when I started, however, I found it a bit more effective to put an adhesive bandage over the mole after the direct application. I would sometimes take a cotton swab and put a drop of apple cider vinegar where the bandage would be touching the mole.

I repeated this process each day, usually sleeping with the bandage at night, and often leaving the bandage on during the day. Occasionally, when I knew I didn't need to go out, I would remove the bandage if the mole, was for no better term, leaking. This would help it dry and it would turn black and pieces would fall off. The bigger the mole the more likely it is to have this reaction.

Repeat and Wait:
My first moles took between six and eight weeks before they were gone. Some moles were gone in just a couple of weeks. I believe my time frames varied because of various reasons. I started to use the emery board instead of poking with the needle, the size of the moles and using the bandages. [See the next section for progress pictures]

For me, the mole would scab over and in the process pieces would come off or just fall off when I would gently rub them. I let this happen as naturally as possible, usually it would happen during the next application of ACV on the cotton pad. Due to the size of the initial moles this went on several times until it got to the bottom. It was dissolving at this point and I would just apply more ACV then cover with a bandage. The mole grew smaller until it was gone. I then let it heal.

I did this to the moles on both sides of my face in the middle of my cheek.

I had one on my eyebrow. I was very careful with this, as I didn't want to drop Apple Cider Vinegar onto my eyelid, let alone my eyeball. I used both the cotton swab and the cotton ball/pad method. (I would soak the cotton swab and just held it against it, making sure not to squeeze with the cotton tip so it wouldn't cause drips.) This method worked better with the cotton swab over the cotton ball or pad. I was very nervous with this one. I had an issue with bandaging over the eyebrow as I didn't want anything in my eye. I did stop the process a little too soon so I may go back and resume the process again.

I did try a mole with only using the vinegar on the bandage but it did not seem to be as effective as using the cotton ball or pad pressed against the skin. It may be because of refreshing the cotton ball or pad during the middle of that 20-minute process or that the cotton ball was able to completely surround the tissue of the mole.

The emery board method, which I started after the first three moles, seemed to be the most effective way to allow the ACV to penetrate the moles. I was able to use the emery board on the tops and sides of the mole and by using the cotton ball or pad it seemed to accelerate the process of getting to the scabbing phase.

I tried not to skip a day and some days I would do two, one in the morning and the other in the evening. For me there was very little pain using this process and typically there was just a stinging sensation when applying the vinegar to the mole.

Images of my mole removal progress

I must warn you the following images are pretty graphic.

These images start with the process of changes to the mole on the right side of my face. One image is with a measuring tape to show the approximate size. I began this process on February 23rd and this was the first mole I attempted to remove. This particular mole I started with the needle poke method. (Next two images)

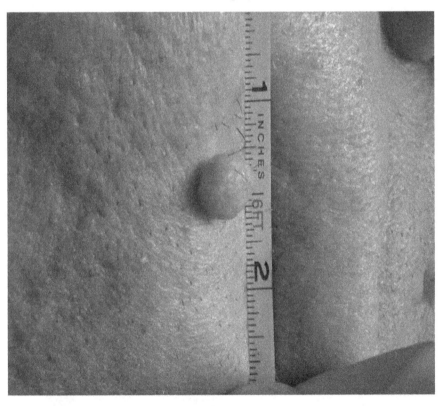

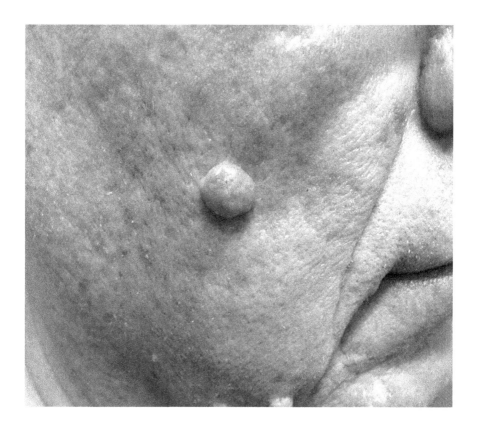

This was an experimental time as it took a while for it to start looking like the image below as I had not used the emery board nor had I poked it at first. When I used the needle I scratched the surface with it and nothing appeared to change so I poked it with the needle and then this started working well and as a result you can see it on the top right image. You can see here just the starting of scabbing happening on the top of the mole.
This was dates March 6 through 11th. (Next five images)
Then more scabbing appeared as I went along.

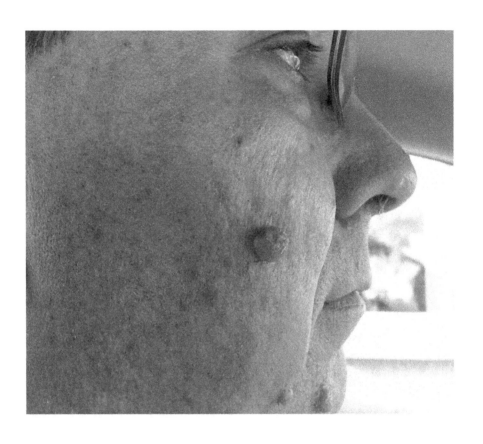

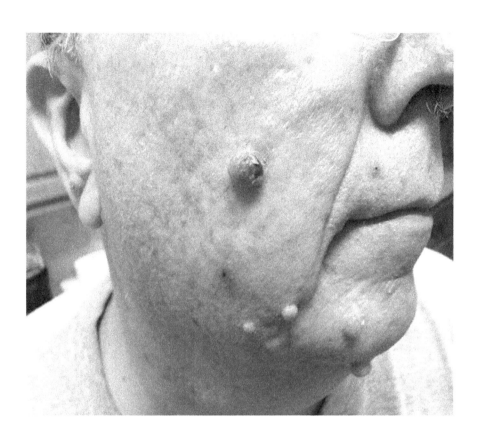

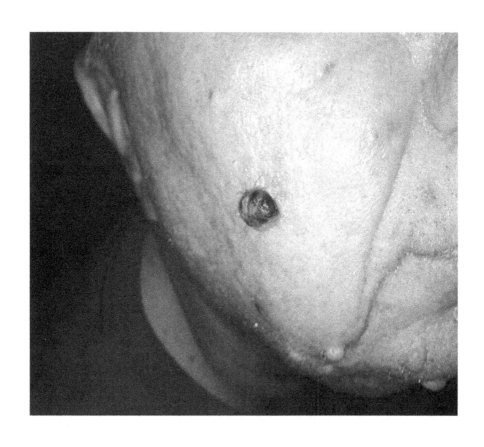

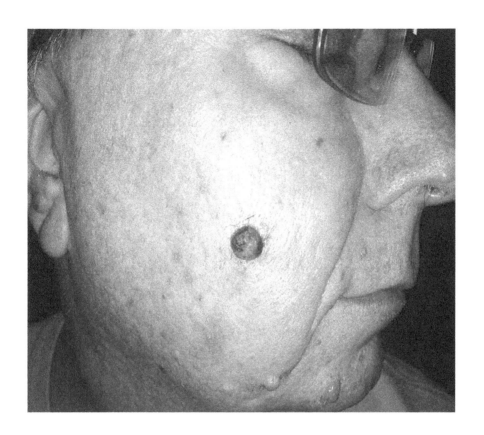

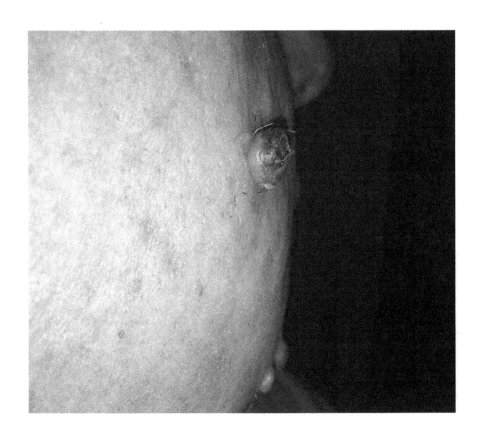

A large piece had dried up and peeled off, I continued to apply the treatment. The following image was taken on March 16th and shows how it has progressed and how much is gone. (Next two images)

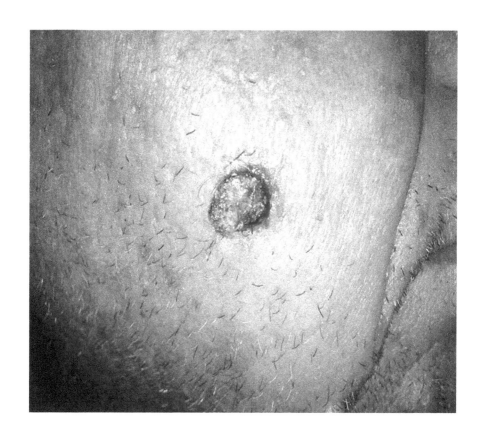

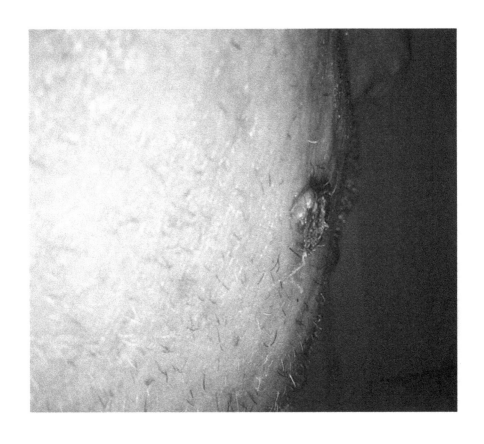

By March 17th the mole had changed to looking like this. Pretty gruesome I know. (Next two images)

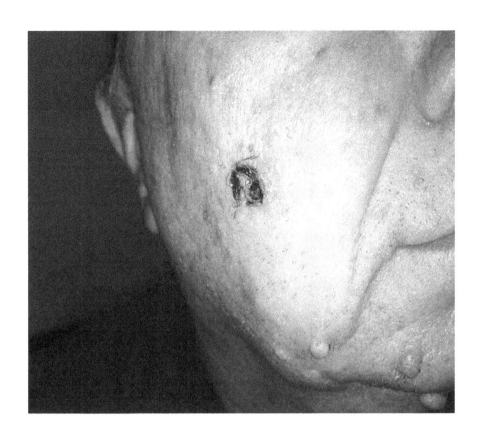

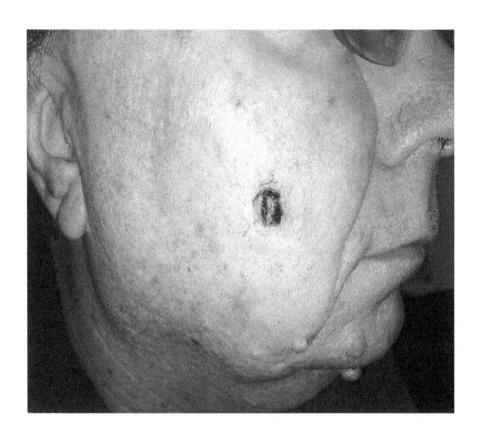

The mole now has continued to shrink as layers peeled away on their own as I applied more ACV. This was on March 19th. (Next two images)

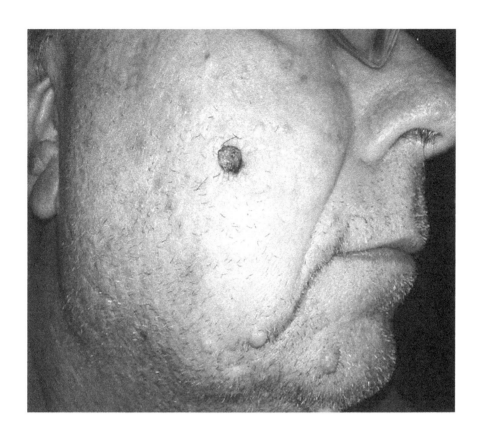

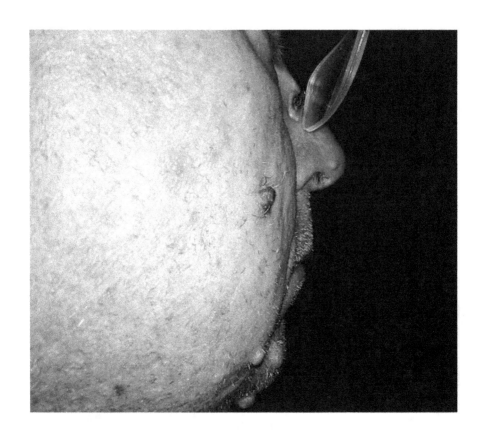

I continued applying, and as you can see it's a little nub sticking out. I did not force pull this off instead I just kept applying. This took until March 26th. (Next Image)

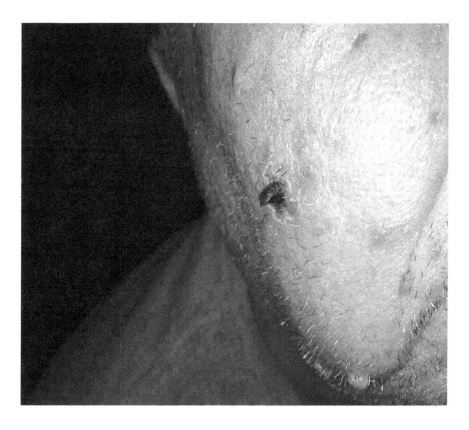

It became much smaller and was nearly gone by the 27th of March. (Next two images)

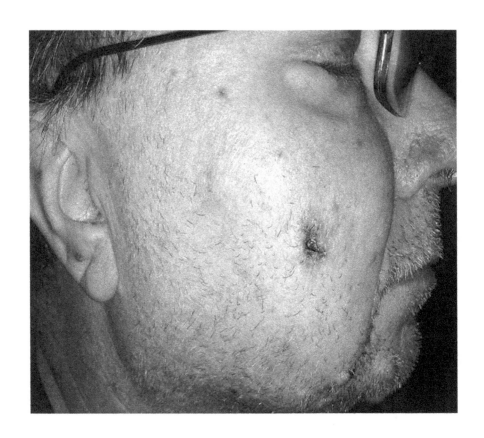

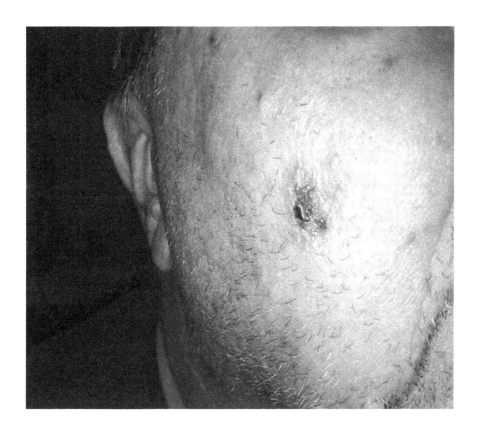

Just a little glob left that after applying the apple cider vinegar application actually wiped away. This was 2 days later on March 29th. (Next two images)

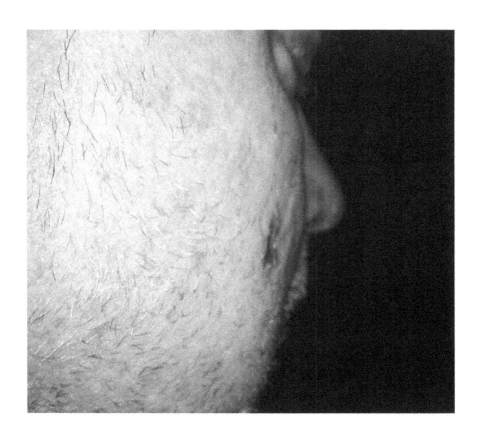

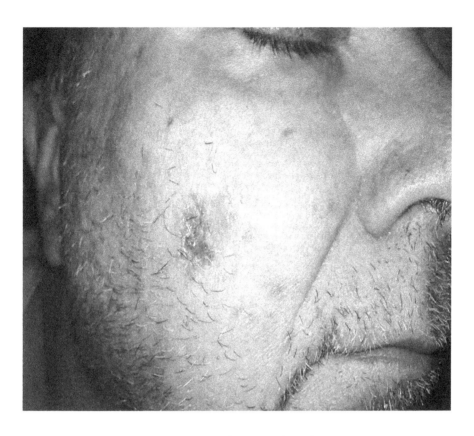

Letting it heal on March 30th.

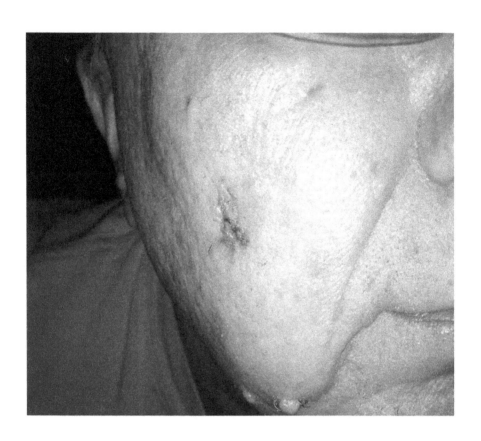

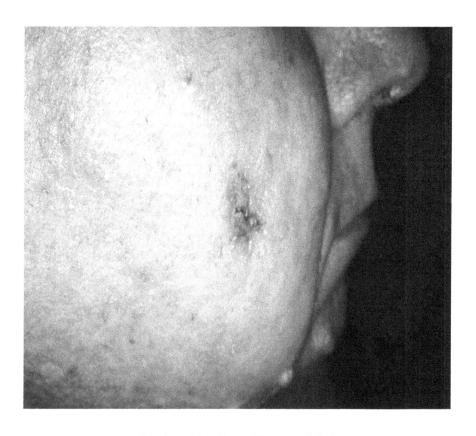

Continued healing still on April 3rd.

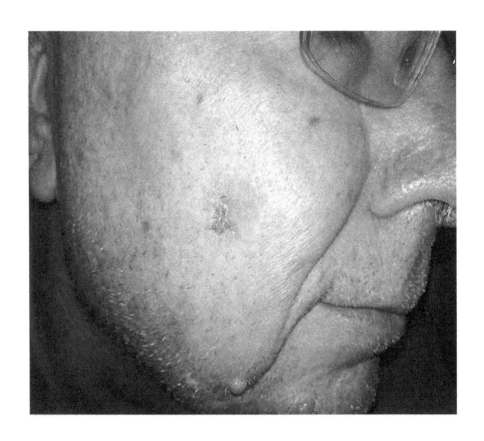

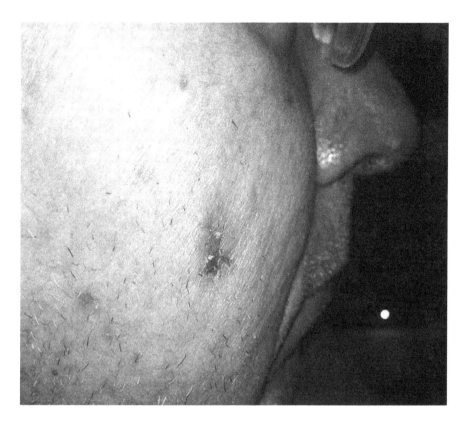

Mole gone, face healed, I had no scar on April 7th.

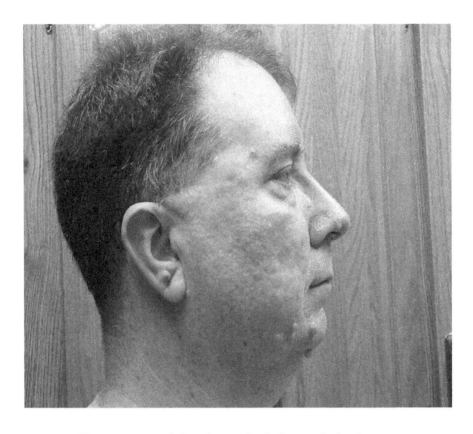

Here are some of the other moles before and after images. Chin and two moles near the right side of my mouth.

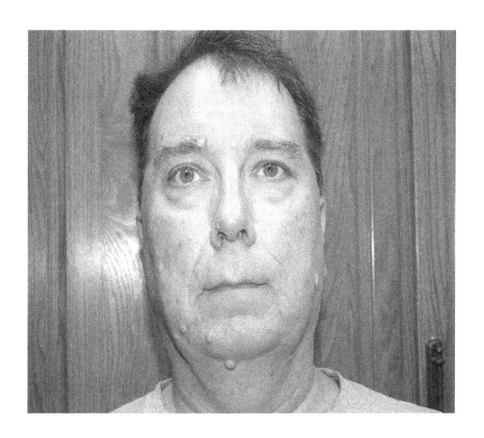

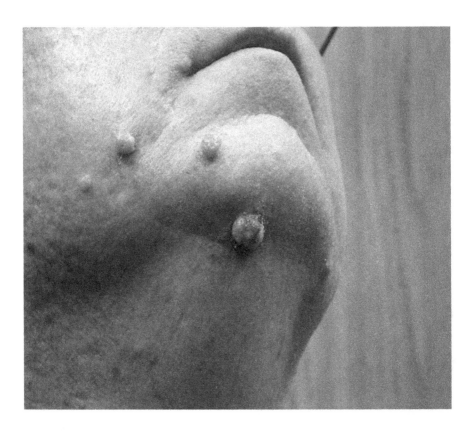

And after!

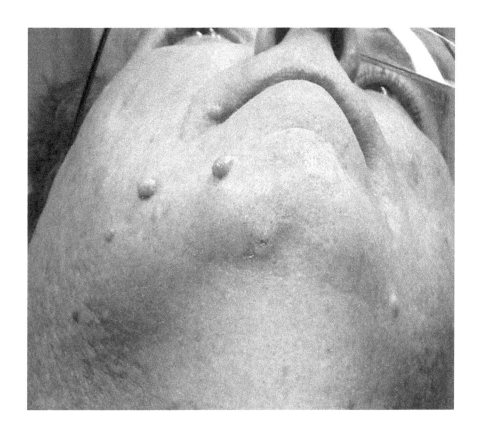

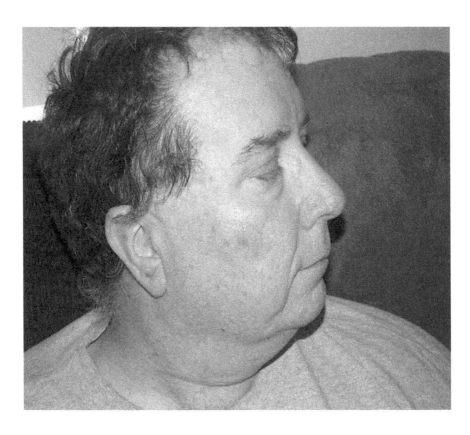

Left side of face mole - before I started.

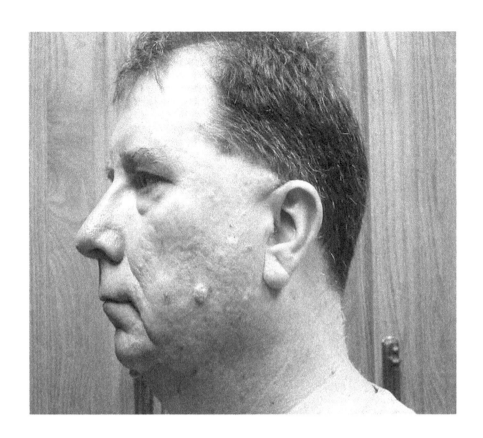

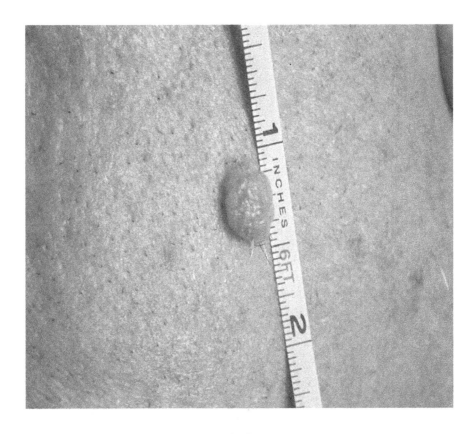

And after!

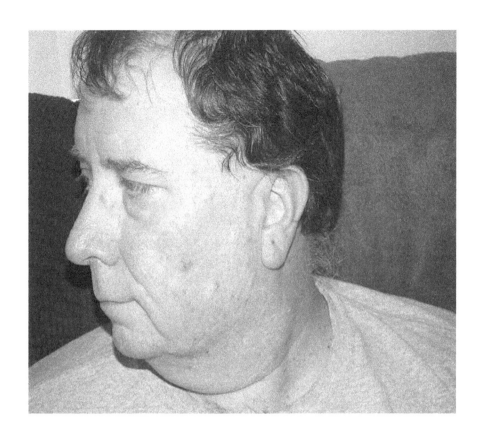

Chapter 5
Some Final Thoughts

Is this the only way to do it? No, there are a number of methods I have researched. I tried many and they didn't work for me, or caused such a disruption that I abandoned them. Some might have worked if I had learned about roughing up the mole first with an emery board instead of trying to scrape or poke them with a thin needle. I think the most amusing or annoying depending on how you look on it—well, more amusing now—annoying at the time was the Oregano oil (an essential oil). The smell was super strong and I tried putting it on each night with an adhesive bandage, but the scent was everywhere and caused us to not be able to sleep at night. Not to mention additional laundry from it getting on pillows, sheets or blankets. It also would not have been good to go to work with this on your face every day due to the pungent aroma.

As I mentioned before I have a ton of moles (100's) all over my body in all kinds of shapes and sizes. I think this was important enough for me to repeat my word of caution in my story. I tried to remove a flat mole that looks like a large freckle and that did not go well. It burned and where I tried to remove it, it instead scarred over.

I had a completely flat black one I started applying coconut oil to and it became raised and lightened in color considerably. I am still in the process of where to go next with this one.

I came across discussions from people who used food grade Hydrogen Peroxide, 35% to apply directly. The only thing is that it will BURN any skin it come into contact with. I am going to approach this with extreme caution.

I have an annoying skin tag behind my knee. I will give you one bit of advice when it comes to skin tags, and that is don't pull on them. I did and my skin tag went from small to large and long.

My journey continues, as I am looking at various methods of dealing with the 100's of moles all over my body in a more effective way. I want to be able to remove the skin tags that I have and hope to share that part of my story as well.

It is too early to speculate on this, but I wanted you to know what I was attempting next, as I still have a lot of other moles. Doing this isn't practical for the sheer number of raised and flat moles that I have.

I wish you the best of luck on your journey.

Printed in the USA
CPSIA information can be obtained
at www.ICGtesting.com
LVHW041606141124
796653LV00011B/280